The PCOS Diet Cookbook For Beginners

A Recipes Guide For Managing PCOS Symptoms Offering Easy Healthy Meal Options To Nourish Your Body

Alycia Heaney

Table of Contents

CHAPTER ONE

Introduction

Polycystic Ovary Syndrome (PCOS) is a complex hormonal disorder primarily affecting people with ovaries. While its exact cause isn't fully understood, it's thought to involve a combination of genetic and environmental factors.

Causes Of PCOS

Hormonal Imbalance: PCOS is associated with an imbalance in reproductive hormones, specifically high levels of androgens (male hormones) like testosterone.

Insulin Resistance: Some individuals with PCOS have insulin resistance, where cells don't respond normally to insulin. This can lead to increased insulin levels, potentially contributing to hormone imbalances.

Genetics: There seems to be a genetic component to PCOS, as it often runs in families.

Symptoms Of PCOS

The symptoms can vary widely between individuals and may include:

Irregular Menstrual Cycles: This is one of the most common signs. Some may have infrequent periods, while others might experience heavy or prolonged bleeding.

Excess Androgen: Manifests as acne, excessive hair growth (hirsutism), or male-pattern baldness.

Polycystic Ovaries: Characterized by enlarged ovaries with small cysts on their outer edges, seen through an ultrasound.

Weight Gain: Many with PCOS struggle with weight gain or find it difficult to lose weight.

Skin Changes: Darkening of skin, particularly along neck creases, in the groin, and underneath breasts due to insulin resistance.

Fertility Issues: Difficulty getting pregnant due to irregular ovulation or lack thereof.

Diagnosis and Management

Diagnosis involves a combination of physical exams, medical history review, blood tests to check hormone levels, and sometimes imaging tests like ultrasounds.

Management typically involves a multi-faceted approach:

Lifestyle Changes: Healthy eating habits, regular exercise, and weight management can help control symptoms, especially those related to insulin resistance.

Medication: Birth control pills, hormone-regulating medications, and medications to address insulin resistance might be prescribed to manage symptoms.

Fertility Treatments: For those struggling with fertility, treatments such as ovulation induction or in vitro fertilization (IVF) may be recommended.

Importance of Diet in Managing PCOS

Diet plays a significant role in managing PCOS symptoms, especially those related to insulin resistance and hormonal imbalances. An effective PCOS diet approach typically focuses on:

Balancing Blood Sugar Levels:

Low Glycemic Index (GI) Foods: These foods cause a slower and steadier rise in blood sugar levels. Opt for whole grains, legumes, fruits, and vegetables.

Balanced Meals: Combining complex carbohydrates with lean protein and healthy fats can help stabilize blood sugar levels.

Managing Weight:

Portion Control: Controlling portion sizes can aid in weight management.

Focusing on Nutrient-Dense Foods: Choose nutrient-rich foods that offer essential vitamins and minerals while being lower in calories.

Healthy Fats: Incorporate sources of healthy fats like avocados, nuts, seeds, and olive oil.

Hormonal Balance:

Fiber-Rich Foods: High-fiber foods can help regulate hormones by aiding in the removal of excess hormones from the body. Include plenty of vegetables, fruits, and whole grains.

Omega-3 Fatty Acids: Found in fatty fish like salmon, as well as flaxseeds and walnuts, they may help in reducing inflammation and supporting hormone balance.

Specific Approaches:

Anti-Inflammatory Foods: Some studies suggest that reducing inflammation can help manage PCOS symptoms. Foods like berries, turmeric, ginger, and green tea possess anti-inflammatory properties.

Dairy and Gluten Consideration: Some individuals with PCOS may benefit from reducing or eliminating dairy and gluten, as these can contribute to inflammation in some cases.

Lifestyle Changes

Regular Physical Activity: Exercise can improve insulin sensitivity and help with weight management, contributing positively to PCOS symptoms.

Stress Management: Stress can impact hormone levels, so practices like yoga, meditation, or mindfulness can be beneficial.

Individualized Approach:

It's important to remember that PCOS varies from person to person, so there isn't a one-size-fits-all diet.

CHAPTER TWO
Polycystic Ovary Syndrome (PCOS)

Polycystic Ovary Syndrome (PCOS) is a hormonal disorder that affects individuals with ovaries, causing a range of symptoms due to hormonal imbalances. It's characterized by:

Hormonal Imbalance:

Androgen Excess: Elevated levels of androgens (male hormones) such as testosterone can lead to symptoms like acne, excessive hair growth, and irregular menstrual cycles.

Insulin Resistance: Some individuals with PCOS experience difficulties in using insulin, leading to higher insulin levels, which can contribute to hormone imbalances.

Impact of Diet on PCOS Symptoms

Blood Sugar Control: Diet can influence insulin levels. Consuming foods with a lower glycemic index can help manage blood sugar levels and reduce insulin resistance.

Weight Management: Since weight gain exacerbates PCOS symptoms, a balanced diet can aid in weight control, reducing the severity of symptoms like irregular periods and androgen excess.

Hormonal Regulation: Certain foods, such as those rich in fiber and omega-3 fatty acids, can help regulate hormone levels, potentially alleviating some PCOS symptoms.

Importance of Healthy Lifestyle Changes

Exercise: Regular physical activity can improve insulin sensitivity, aid in weight management, and alleviate PCOS symptoms.

Stress Management: Stress can worsen hormone imbalances. Adopting stress-reducing practices like meditation, yoga, or mindfulness can positively impact symptoms.

Sleep: Quality sleep is crucial for overall health and can influence hormone regulation and weight management, both significant factors in managing PCOS.

Nutritional Guidelines for PCOS Management

Understanding the PCOS diet involves specific nutritional guidelines aimed at managing symptoms and hormonal imbalances. Here are key points to consider:

Complex Carbohydrates: Opt for whole grains, legumes, fruits, and vegetables to regulate blood sugar levels due to their lower glycemic index.

Lean Protein: Include sources like poultry, fish, tofu, legumes, and lean cuts of meat to support muscle health and help stabilize blood sugar levels.

Healthy Fats: Incorporate sources of monounsaturated and polyunsaturated fats such as avocados, nuts, seeds, and olive oil, as they support hormone production and overall health.

Fiber-Rich Foods: High-fiber foods aid in hormone regulation and include vegetables, fruits, whole grains, and legumes.

Balancing Macronutrients for Hormonal Health

Proteins: Assist in building and repairing tissues, including hormone production and regulation.

Fats: Essential for hormone synthesis and maintenance. Omega-3 fatty acids, in particular, have anti-inflammatory properties.

Carbohydrates: Focus on complex carbohydrates that digest more slowly, preventing sudden spikes in blood sugar levels.

Foods to Limit or Avoid with PCOS

Highly Processed Foods: These often contain added sugars and unhealthy fats, contributing to weight gain and exacerbating insulin resistance.

Sugary Foods and Beverages: Sodas, candies, pastries, and other high-sugar items can spike blood sugar levels and aggravate insulin resistance.

Refined Carbohydrates: White bread, white rice, and sugary cereals should be limited due to their higher glycemic index.

Trans Fats: Found in many processed and fried foods, Trans fats can increase inflammation and insulin resistance.

Excessive Dairy and Gluten: Some individuals may benefit from reducing or eliminating these items, as they can trigger inflammation in certain cases. However, this varies among individuals and should be discussed with a healthcare professional.

Meal Planning for PCOS

Planning PCOS-friendly meals involves creating balanced, nutrient-dense menus that support hormonal health and help manage symptoms. Here are some tips and a sample meal plan to get started:

Balance Macronutrients: Each meal should ideally contain a combination of lean protein, healthy fats, and complex carbohydrates to stabilize blood sugar levels.

Portion Control: Be mindful of portion sizes to prevent overeating and support weight management.

Include Fiber: Aim for high-fiber foods like vegetables, fruits, whole grains, and legumes to regulate hormones and aid digestion.

Choose Low-Glycemic Index Foods: Opt for whole grains, such as quinoa or brown rice, over refined grains like white rice or pasta.

Healthy Snacking: Plan nutritious snacks like nuts, Greek yogurt, veggies with hummus, or fruit to maintain

energy levels between meals.

CHAPTER THREE
Sample Meal Plan

Breakfast:

- Greek yogurt parfait with berries and almonds

- Whole grain toast with avocado and poached eggs

Lunch:

- Grilled chicken or tofu salad with mixed greens, veggies, and a drizzle of olive oil and balsamic vinegar

- Quinoa and black bean stuffed bell peppers

Snack:

- Apple slices with almond butter

- Carrot sticks with hummus

Dinner:

- Baked salmon or tempeh with roasted vegetables (broccoli, cauliflower, carrots)

- Brown rice or sweet potato

Portion Control:

- Protein: A palm-sized portion (about 3–4 ounces) of chicken, fish, or tofu.

- Carbohydrates: 1/2 to 1 cup of cooked whole grains or legumes.

- Healthy Fats: A tablespoon of olive oil, a handful of nuts or seeds.

- Vegetables: Fill half of your plate with non-starchy vegetables.

High-Fiber and Protein-Packed Breakfast Ideas

Some energizing breakfast options that are high in fiber, packed with protein, and suitable for individuals managing PCOS:

Greek Yogurt Parfait:

- Layer Greek yogurt with mixed berries (like raspberries,

blueberries, or strawberries) and a sprinkle of nuts or seeds for added protein and fiber.

Vegetable Omelette:

- Make an omelette with spinach, tomatoes, bell peppers, and a sprinkle of feta or goat cheese for added flavor.

Quinoa Breakfast Bowl:

- Cook quinoa in almond milk, then top it with sliced bananas, chopped nuts, and a drizzle of honey or maple syrup.

Chia Seed Pudding:

- Mix chia seeds with almond milk, a dash of vanilla extract, and a sweetener like honey or stevia. Let it sit overnight and top it with fresh fruit in the morning.

Smoothie Bowl:

- Blend spinach, frozen berries, a banana, Greek yogurt, and a splash of almond milk. Top it with granola, nuts, and seeds for added crunch and nutrients.

Avocado Toast with Egg:

- Mash avocado on whole grain toast and top it with a poached or fried egg. Sprinkle some red pepper flakes for a kick.

PCOS-Friendly Smoothies:

Berry Blast Smoothie: Blend mixed berries, spinach, Greek yogurt, almond milk, and a scoop of protein powder or chia seeds for an extra protein boost.

Green Goddess Smoothie: Combine spinach, kale, banana, avocado, almond milk, and a scoop of hemp seeds or nut butter for healthy fats and protein.

Tips for PCOS-Friendly Breakfasts

Fiber Focus: Incorporate ingredients like berries, chia seeds, flaxseeds, and whole grains to boost fiber intake.

Protein Power: Include sources like Greek yogurt, eggs, nuts, seeds, and protein powder for a satisfying and protein-packed meal.

Complex Carbohydrates: Opt for whole grains like oats, quinoa, or whole grain bread to maintain stable blood sugar levels.

Experimenting with these recipes can provide variety and ensure a nutritious start to the day, promoting energy levels and helping manage PCOS symptoms effectively. Adjust ingredients to suit personal preferences and dietary needs while keeping the focus on nutrient density and balance.

Lunchtime Favorites (Nutrient-Rich Lunch Ideas)

Some nutrient-rich lunch ideas that include salads, wraps, and grain bowls, perfect for sustaining energy levels and supporting those managing PCOS:

Quinoa and Veggie Salad:

- Mix cooked quinoa with a variety of colorful vegetables like bell peppers, cucumbers, cherry tomatoes, and add in some chickpeas or grilled chicken for protein. Toss with a lemon vinaigrette.

Mediterranean Chickpea Salad:

- Combine chickpeas with diced cucumber, red onion, olives, and feta cheese. Dress it with olive oil, lemon juice, and fresh herbs like parsley or mint.

Grilled Chicken Wrap:

- Fill a whole grain wrap with grilled chicken, avocado, lettuce, and a spread of hummus. Roll it up for a satisfying meal.

Sushi-Inspired Quinoa Bowl:

- Mix cooked quinoa with cucumber, avocado slices, shredded carrots, and cooked edamame. Drizzle with a light soy-sesame dressing.

Veggie Stir-Fry with Brown Rice:

- Stir-fry mixed vegetables like broccoli, bell peppers, snap peas, and tofu or shrimp. Serve it over brown rice with a light soy-ginger

sauce.

CHAPTER FOUR

Recipes to Sustain Energy Levels

Protein-Packed Salad: Incorporate lean proteins like grilled chicken, turkey, tofu, or beans into salads to keep you feeling full and satisfied.

Healthy Fats: Add sources of healthy fats like avocado, nuts, seeds, or a drizzle of olive oil to provide lasting energy and aid in nutrient absorption.

Whole Grains: Opt for whole grain options like quinoa, brown rice, or whole grain wraps to provide complex carbohydrates for sustained energy.

PCOS-Friendly Tips

Colorful Veggies: Load up on colorful vegetables for a variety of nutrients and antioxidants.

Balanced Meals: Aim for a mix of lean protein, healthy fats, fiber, and complex carbs for a well-rounded and satisfying lunch.

Portion Control: Be mindful of portions to prevent overeating and support weight management, a key factor in managing PCOS symptoms.

These lunch ideas not only provide essential nutrients but also offer a balance of macronutrients to sustain energy levels throughout the day. Feel free to customize these recipes according to personal preferences while keeping a focus on nutrient density and balance.

Healthy Snack Options for PCOS Management

Snacks play a significant role in managing hunger, stabilizing blood sugar levels, and satisfying cravings, especially for individuals managing PCOS. Here are some healthy snack options and strategies:

Mixed Nuts and Seeds: A handful of almonds, walnuts, or pumpkin seeds provide healthy fats and protein to keep you full.

Greek Yogurt with Berries: Greek yogurt is high in protein and pairs well with antioxidant-rich berries.

Hummus and Veggies: Carrot sticks, cucumber slices, or bell pepper strips dipped in hummus make a satisfying and nutritious snack.

Hard-Boiled Eggs: A convenient and protein-rich snack that can be prepared in advance.

Apple Slices with Nut Butter: Apples provide fiber while nut butter offers healthy fats and protein.

Air-Popped Popcorn: A whole-grain snack when prepared without excess butter or oil can satisfy cravings for something crunchy.

Managing Cravings and Sudden Hunger Pangs

Mindful Eating: Listen to your body's hunger cues and eat when you're genuinely hungry rather than in response to emotions or external cues.

Hydration: Sometimes thirst can be mistaken for hunger. Stay hydrated by drinking water or herbal teas throughout the day.

Balanced Snacks: Aim for snacks that combine protein, healthy fats, and fiber to help keep you satisfied until the next meal.

Portable Snacks for On-the-Go Days

Trail Mix: Create a mix of nuts, seeds, dried fruits, and a few dark chocolate pieces for a portable and energizing snack.

Protein Bars: Look for bars with minimal added sugars and higher protein content for a quick on-the-go option.

String Cheese or Cheese Cubes: Pair them with whole grain crackers for a balanced snack.

Fruit: Apples, bananas, or oranges are convenient and portable choices that provide natural sugars and fiber.

PCOS-Friendly Snack Tips

Preparation is Key: Plan and prepare snacks in advance to have them readily available when hunger strikes.

Avoid Highly Processed Snacks: Opt for whole foods instead of highly processed snacks with added sugars and unhealthy fats.

Portion Control: Be mindful of portion sizes, especially with calorie-dense snacks, to maintain a healthy weight.

By choosing nutrient-dense snacks and being mindful of hunger cues, individuals managing PCOS can effectively manage cravings, keep energy levels stable, and support overall health and well-being. Adjust these snack options to suit personal preferences and dietary needs while focusing on a balance of nutrients.

Balanced Dinner Recipes for PCOS

Some balanced dinner recipes tailored for individuals managing PCOS, including one-pot meals and easy weeknight dinners that incorporate PCOS-friendly ingredients:

Sheet Pan Chicken and Vegetables:

- Marinate chicken breasts in a mix of olive oil, lemon juice, and herbs. Roast them with a variety of vegetables like broccoli, bell peppers, and sweet potatoes on a sheet pan for a flavorful and nutrient-rich meal.

Quinoa and Black Bean Stuffed Peppers:

- Hollow out bell peppers and stuff them with a mix of cooked quinoa, black beans, diced tomatoes, corn, and spices. Bake until the peppers are tender and serve with a side salad.

Salmon or Tofu Stir-Fry:

- Stir-fry salmon or tofu with mixed vegetables like broccoli, snap peas, carrots, and bell peppers. Flavor it with a soy-ginger sauce and serve over brown rice or quinoa.

Turkey or Lentil Bolognese:

- Cook ground turkey or lentils with onions, garlic, tomatoes, and herbs to make a hearty sauce. Serve it over whole grain pasta or zucchini noodles for a low-carb option.

CHAPTER FIVE

One-Pot Meals and Easy Weeknight Dinners

Vegetable Curry with Chickpeas:

- Simmer chickpeas, mixed vegetables, and diced tomatoes in a coconut milk-based curry sauce with spices like turmeric, cumin, and coriander. Serve it with brown rice or quinoa.

Lemon Garlic Shrimp or Tofu Pasta:

- Sauté shrimp or tofu with garlic, lemon zest, and spinach. Toss it with whole grain pasta and a touch of olive oil for a simple yet satisfying dinner.

Vegetable and Lentil Soup:

- Simmer lentils, assorted vegetables, vegetable broth, and herbs in a pot for a comforting and nutrient-packed soup.

Incorporating PCOS-Friendly Ingredients

Lean Proteins: Choose lean sources like poultry, fish, tofu, or legumes for protein without excessive saturated fats.

Whole Grains: Opt for whole grains such as quinoa, brown rice, or whole grain pasta for fiber and complex carbohydrates.

Colorful Veggies: Include a variety of colorful vegetables for a wide range of nutrients and antioxidants.

PCOS-Friendly Dinner Tips

Meal Prep: Prepare ingredients in advance to streamline dinner preparation, especially on busy weekdays.

Cooking Methods: Focus on healthier cooking methods like baking, grilling, steaming, or sautéing instead of frying to reduce added fats.

Creating balanced dinners involves incorporating nutrient-dense ingredients that support overall health and help manage PCOS symptoms. Feel free to modify these recipes based on personal preferences and dietary needs while focusing on a balance of macronutrients and wholesome ingredients.

Desserts and Treats

Managing PCOS doesn't mean skipping out on desserts entirely. Here are some indulgent yet PCOS-approved dessert options, healthy sweet treats, and sugar alternatives for occasional indulgence:

Dark Chocolate-Covered Berries:

- Dip strawberries, blueberries, or raspberries in melted dark chocolate (70% cocoa or higher) for a sweet treat with antioxidants.

Chia Seed Pudding with Fruit:

- Create chia seed pudding using almond milk, a touch of honey or stevia, and top it with sliced fruits like mango, berries, or kiwi.

Baked Apples with Cinnamon:

- Core apples and bake them with a sprinkle of cinnamon and a touch of honey. Serve with a dollop of Greek yogurt.

Frozen Banana Bites:

- Slice bananas, dip them in Greek yogurt, and then freeze. Optionally, roll them in crushed nuts or dark chocolate before freezing for added flavor.

Healthy Sweet Options for Occasional Treats

Fruit Sorbet:

- Blend frozen fruits like mango, pineapple, or berries with a touch of lemon juice for a refreshing and naturally sweet sorbet.

Homemade Granola Bars:

- Make your own granola bars using oats, nuts, seeds, and a touch of honey or dates for sweetness.

Greek Yogurt Parfait:

- Layer Greek yogurt with sliced fruits, nuts, and a drizzle of honey or a sprinkle of cinnamon for a satisfying dessert.

Sugar Alternatives and Dessert Hacks

Stevia or Monk Fruit: Consider using natural sugar substitutes like stevia or monk fruit in moderation to sweeten desserts without spiking blood sugar levels.

Healthy Baking Substitutes: Use mashed bananas, unsweetened applesauce, or dates as natural sweeteners in baking recipes instead of refined sugars.

Portion Control: Enjoy desserts in moderation, focusing on smaller portions to satisfy cravings without overindulging.

PCOS-Friendly Dessert Tips

Nutrient-Dense Ingredients: Incorporate nuts, seeds, fruits, and Greek yogurt into desserts to add nutrients and balance out sweetness.

Experiment with Flavors: Enhance desserts with natural flavorings like vanilla extract, citrus zest, or spices such as cinnamon or nutmeg for added taste without added sugar.

DIY Desserts: Making desserts at home allows you to control ingredients, sweetness, and portion sizes.

Balancing occasional treats with nutrient-dense ingredients and mindful portion control allows individuals managing PCOS to enjoy desserts without compromising their health goals. Experiment with different recipes and ingredients to find satisfying sweet options that work well for personal preferences and dietary needs.

Lifestyle and Dietary Tips

Lifestyle and dietary factors beyond food choices play significant roles in managing PCOS effectively:

Importance of Exercise in PCOS Management:

Improved Insulin Sensitivity: Regular exercise helps increase insulin sensitivity, reducing insulin resistance often associated with PCOS.

Weight Management: Physical activity aids in weight control, which is crucial for managing PCOS symptoms, especially those related to hormonal balance and fertility.

Hormonal Regulation: Exercise can help regulate hormone levels, potentially reducing androgen excess and improving menstrual regularity.

CHAPTER SIX

Stress Management Techniques

Mindfulness and Meditation: Practicing mindfulness and meditation can reduce stress levels, which in turn can positively impact hormone balance.

Yoga or Tai Chi: These practices combine movement with relaxation techniques, offering physical benefits while reducing stress.

Breathing Exercises: Deep breathing exercises can activate the body's relaxation response, helping to manage stress.

Sleep and Its Role in Hormonal Health

Hormonal Regulation: Quality sleep is crucial for hormone regulation, including those involved in PCOS management. Lack of sleep can disrupt hormonal balance, potentially exacerbating symptoms.

Stress Reduction: Adequate sleep supports stress management, as it allows the body to recover and recharge, reducing overall stress levels.

Healthy Sleep Hygiene: Establishing a consistent sleep schedule, creating a relaxing bedtime routine, and optimizing sleep environment contribute to better sleep quality.

Incorporating These Tips into Daily Life

Consistency: Regular exercise, stress management techniques, and good sleep habits work best when practiced consistently.

Personalized Approach: Find activities that resonate with you individually to ensure long-term commitment and success.

Seek Support: Consider joining support groups or seeking guidance from healthcare professionals specializing in PCOS management for personalized advice.

Addressing lifestyle factors like exercise, stress management, and sleep hygiene in addition to dietary changes can significantly impact PCOS symptoms. Integrating these practices into daily life may require patience and experimentation to find what works best for individual needs. Prioritizing a balanced approach to overall wellness can aid in effectively managing PCOS and supporting long-term health.

PCOS Diet and Beyond

Long-term strategies for managing PCOS involve adopting sustainable lifestyle changes, including a balanced diet and beyond:

Long-Term Strategies for PCOS Management:

Consistent Exercise: Regular physical activity supports hormonal balance, weight management, and overall well-being. Aim for a mix of cardio, strength training, and flexibility exercises.

Stress Management: Incorporate stress-reducing practices like meditation, yoga, or deep breathing exercises into your routine to support hormonal health.

Quality Sleep: Prioritize good sleep hygiene by establishing a regular sleep schedule and creating a relaxing bedtime routine for better hormone regulation.

Regular Check-Ups: Schedule regular check-ups with healthcare professionals specializing in PCOS to monitor symptoms and make necessary adjustments to your management plan.

Encouragement for a Sustainable PCOS Diet

Focus on Progress, Not Perfection: Embrace gradual changes and celebrate small victories in your journey towards a healthier lifestyle.

Flexibility and Balance: Allow for occasional indulgences while maintaining a predominantly nutrient-dense diet. Balance is key for long-term sustainability.

Experiment and Adapt: Use various foods and recipes that work well for you. Adapt your diet based on what makes you feel best and fits your lifestyle.

Seek Support: Connect with support groups, online communities, or healthcare professionals specializing in PCOS to find encouragement, advice, and motivation.

Overall Approach:

Consistency Over Time: Sustainable changes take time to yield noticeable results. Stay consistent with healthy habits, even during setbacks.

Mindful Eating: Focus on mindful eating practices, paying attention to hunger and fullness cues, and choosing nourishing foods most of the time.

Self-Compassion: Be kind to yourself throughout the process. Managing PCOS is a journey, and setbacks are natural. Practice self-compassion and patience.

Creating a sustainable PCOS management plan involves a holistic approach that encompasses diet, exercise, stress management, and overall wellness. Embrace lifestyle changes gradually, seeking support and guidance when needed, to ensure a sustainable and successful long-term approach to managing PCOS.

Conclusion

Managing PCOS involves a multifaceted approach that goes beyond diet, encompassing lifestyle adjustments and self-care practices. By focusing on a balanced diet rich in nutrient-dense foods, incorporating regular exercise, managing stress, prioritizing quality sleep, and seeking support from healthcare professionals, individuals can effectively manage PCOS symptoms and support overall well-being.

Remember, there's no one-size-fits-all solution. Personalized approaches tailored to individual needs and preferences are key. Embrace gradual changes, celebrate progress, and maintain a positive mindset throughout the journey. With consistency, patience, and self-compassion, sustainable management of PCOS is achievable.

Seeking support from healthcare professionals, connecting with communities, and implementing long-term strategies can pave the way toward a healthier and fulfilling life while managing PCOS. Keep focusing on overall health and well-being, and remember, you're not alone in this journey.

THE END